The Alzheimer's Journey

Early On-Set

Mild Stage

Late Stage

Moderate Stage

Connecting the Puzzle Pieces

Early On-Set Stage

Seminar Workbook

By: Mr. Roy Peet Poillon
Ms. Marie Ann Raccuia, RN

This workbook is about uniting the family around a loved one with Alzheimer's disease.

It is a companion to The Alzheimer's Journey, Connecting the Puzzle Pieces Seminar. The attendee is required to use this workbook as a guide to the presentation. The work assignments in this book are designed to assist the attendee in learning more about specific subject areas.

First Edition: June, 2018

Printed in the United States of America

ISBN: 978-0-9973482-6-2

Table of Content

INTRODUCTION: Unifying the Alzheimer's Family

In the Alzheimer's journey a great deal of effort, compassion and commitment will be required from each family member. The demands of this disease are relentless and will not be ignored nor can they be pushed to the side. This journey is best traveled as a unified family. In the Alzheimer's journey there are 7 dynamics known to take place. Each Alzheimer's family will experience these dynamics and each dynamic "needs to be identified". The key is to understand and use these dynamics as a tool, to access the four primary support structures. In this seminar, "The Alzheimer's Journey Connecting the Puzzle Pieces" will show how to connect the 7 dynamics to the 4 primary support structures.

In the Alzheimer's journey:
1. The families core values will be challenged, our values motivate us to see things through.
2. Knowledge of the disease is required, what is Alzheimer's, how does it progress.
3. The ability to make effective, informed, proactive decisions is required. (there will be many decisions).
4. Facing the critical issues that present in each stage of diminishment, (each stage has its own critical issues).
5. How to managing dementia related behavior, this knowledge will be a valuable survival skill for the family.
6. Using spiritual faith practices, will give respite and strength, courage and hope.
7. Roles and responsibility are assigned to each member of the family.

This is complicated and the sooner your family gets educated, united and organized, the better.

As the pieces are connected a clearer picture will develop. The first piece is critical, it is the starting point; the 7 Dynamics in an Alzheimer's Family outlines what a family will experience and needs to know or do, prior to it happening. The next piece is where the family can turn for support. Here they will find four primary support structures. It is critical to understand both; what will happen (7 Dynamics), where to go for help (4 Primary Support Structures).

The First Assignment, (view On-Line): Please watch the recommended videos prior to starting the seminar.

www.youtube.com   search UCLA Alzheimer's and Dementia Care Program Introduction.

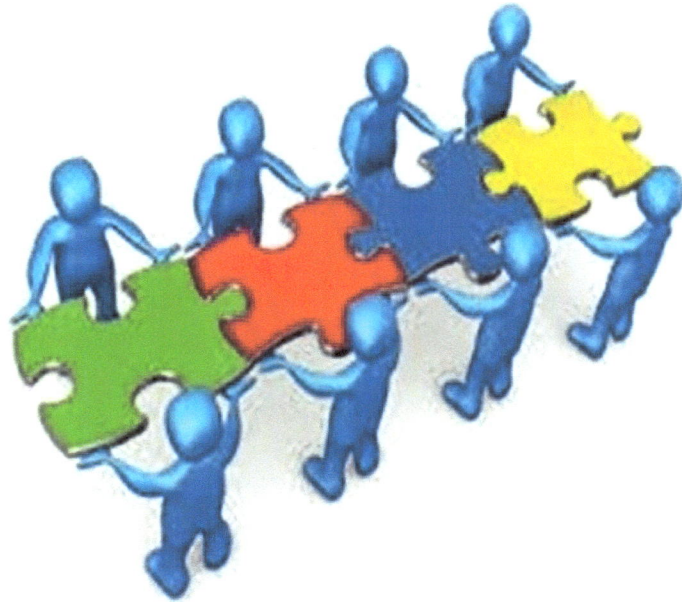

SESSION ONE

Connecting 7 Dynamics with the 4 Primary Support Structures

7 Dynamics in an Alzheimer's Family Model

A family needs to gain an insight as to how these 7 dynamics can be used to their advantage. The 7 Dynamics in an Alzheimer's Family is the most effective model to use when seeking assistance from the 4 primary support structures. The goal is to help the family get the most out of the 4 Primary support structures.

To follow are the 7 Dynamics in an Alzheimer's Family. This outline will help the reader understand how they connect to each other and how they can help the family.

The dynamics begin with an examination of the family core values and ends with roles and responsibilities. The in-between dynamics are some of the things that a family will experience, which they can prepare for in advance.

The 7 Dynamics in an Alzheimer's Family Model:

1. Family Core Values

2. The Disease, How it progresses

3. Family Decisions Making Model

4. Facing The Critical Issues

5. Managing Dementia Related Behavior

6. Spiritual Faith Practices

7. Roles and Responsibilities

The 4 Primary Support Structures

The family cannot go through the Alzheimer's journey alone. They will require extensive support during their loved ones decline. This support will come from four primary resources. Unfortunately, there is no one single resource structure that provides all four.

Each resource is its own structure. These structures don't talk to each other, they don't collaborate unless within the same health system. In many cases accessing these structure can be very challenging. The problem is many of these resources do not understand the families holistic needs. They are set up to provide services, but not necessarily for the exact needs of this type of family. Because of the support structure complexity, and the resources lack of understanding, it is best to use a model that can extract what the family needs from each resource.

4 Primary Support Structures

1. **The Family Support Structure:** The family members are their own resource support structure as they support the primary caregiver and loved one.
2. **The Church Support Structure:** The church is a resource support structure for the family members, primary caregiver and loved one.
3. **The Community Support Structure:** The community (professional services, medical, govt agencies and non for profits) is a support structure for the family members, primary caregiver and loved one.
4. **The Employer Support Structure:** The employer is a support structure for the primary caregiver.

The reason accessing the Four Primary Support Structures presents a problem is because they do not automatically show up at your front door. They offer services and leave it up to you to find them. In this single 7 session seminar each dynamic will be explained in detail. The goal is for the family to use these dynamics each time they access one of the 4 Primary Support Structures. By using this model the family will approach each structure in a united, organized and proactive way to ensure the best outcome.

When accessing one of the Four Structures, the family members and primary caregiver will use the 7 Dynamics in an Alzheimer's Family as a check list, (did we do this?) to ensure all points were covered.

For Example: The family is facing a critical issue, they need to access a "Community Support Structure" in this case "moving their loved one into a memory care facility".

Dynamic One: Family Core Values. The family determined safety of their loved one was a family value. Also, quality of daily living. A memory care facility in this situation meets both values.

Dynamic Two: Understand the disease. How it progresses. Which of the 8 thinking skills has declined and will this behavior worsen as the disease progresses?

Dynamic Three: Family Decision Making Model. The model is used so everyone's input is included whereby an effective and informed decision is made.

Dynamic Four: Facing Critical Issues. Often there are more than just one critical issues when trying to create a solution. Facing all the known issues is important because one may impact the outcome of the other.

Dynamic Five: Managing Dementia Related Behavior. What are the behaviors being observed and how well are they being managed? Will they be better managed in a facility?

Dynamic Six: Spiritual Faith Practices. Are we asking for God's Will to guide us?

Dynamic Seven: Roles and Responsibility. For the assigned "financial role and responsibility", this person calculates and provides input on the financial aspects of the decision. The same is true for those assigned to other roles. Everyone's involvement has an assigned responsibility to participate.

By using the 7 Dynamics model in accessing this phase of the Alzheimer's journey a family has more effectively included a way to respond, in a process whereby everyone is united and their shared gifts are included.

Be Flexible: There is a metamorphic shift in each family member during this journey. Be understanding of each other, because each will choose their own path in how they will deal with this journey. Uniting everyone's individual journey, is a part of the family experience in Alzheimer's.

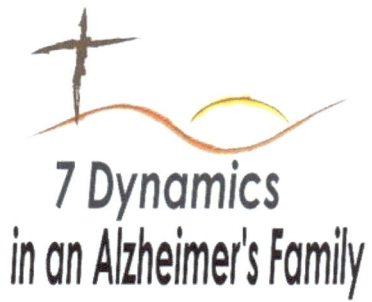

**7 Dynamics
in an Alzheimer's Family**

1st Dynamic

Family Core Values

Plain and simple; Family Core Values is what brings everything together; the "7 Dynamics in an Alzheimer's Family with the 4 Primary Support Structures". That is why the Family Core Values is the first of the 7 Dynamics in the Alzheimer's journey. It is what will be impacted first, and its effect lasts throughout the entire journey.

Before we begin, let's get the most important insight identified and agreed too. The family will need to know who they are, what guides them as a family and how is this awareness helpful in the Alzheimer's Journey? Each family member needs to take a moment and complete the below questions for themselves. First we are individuals, then we are members of the family.

Who are we as individuals? This question should be answered before we start in order to combine the members of the family . If you are going to ask yourself to make changes, then it is best to understand, "Change from What"?

I Am these things / I Do these things: (short description, what are your primary roles in life?)

_____
_____
_____

I Feel this way about myself and my accomplishments: (short description)

_____
_____
_____

What do I want to be doing in the future (short description)

_____
_____
_____

Plain and Simple, using the 7 Dynamics brings everything together. But it is the Family Core Values that allow it to work.

In Values, we find ourselves taking a stance on how we will follow a certain way towards making a decision. It is therefore important to understand the family core values, prior to making critical decisions about the lives of our family members and loved one. This is titled, "**Value Based Decision Making**".

Exercise # One

Complete this form by writing your understanding of the top three core values then present them to the family. Each family member takes their turn. (no opinions should be given, just listen)

1.

2.

3.

When everyone has spoken, write down the top three that are common values between all individual family members:

1.

2.

3.

Exercise # Two:

Use the above list to rank "*by prioritizing*" the three common values, choose your top two family values, which are most important to everyone.

1.

2.

Exercise # Three:

From this list, You now have your top two core family values, which represents what is most important to your family. You will use your Family Core Values in every part of this journey.

OUR FAMILY VALUES ARE:

_____
_____
_____

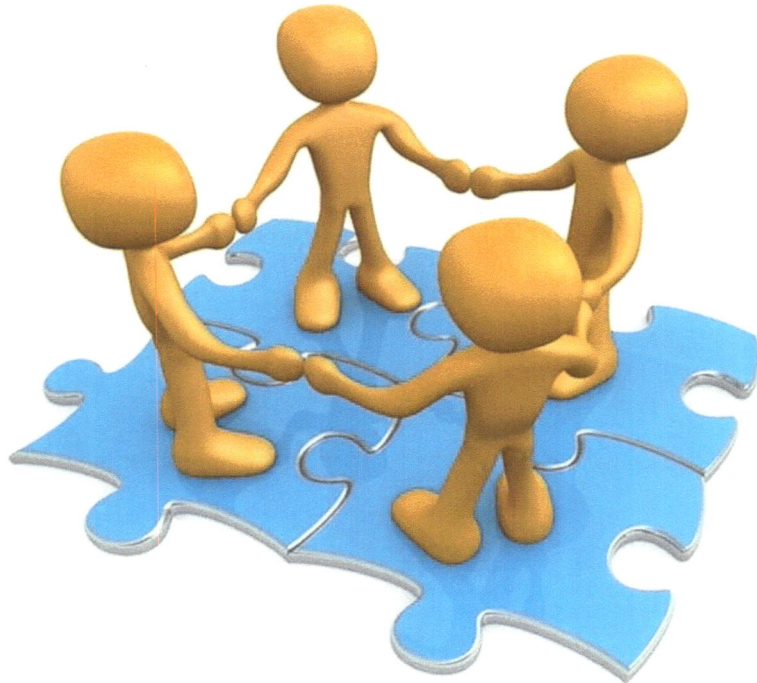

Session Two

Connecting the Disease with its Disease Progression

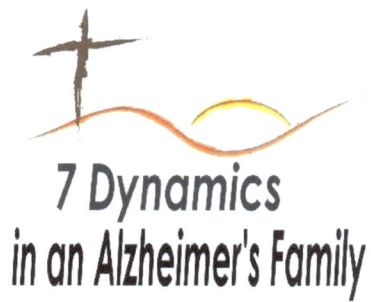

7 Dynamics
in an Alzheimer's Family

2nd Dynamic

Understanding the Disease

There are Six steps a family will take to better understand the Alzheimer's Disease journey.

Steps:

1. How the Brain Works
2. Find a Specialist
3. Get an Appointment
4. Get an Assessment
5. Get a Diagnosis
6. Understand How Alzheimer's Progresses

First Understand Dementia

1. Dementia is a condition or syndrome, (it in itself is not a disease).
2. Alzheimer's Disease is the disease that causes dementia. There are 70+ diseases that have dementia like symptoms.
3. In 80% of dementia patients, Alzheimer's Disease is the diagnosed disease.

Alzheimer's Disease is a disease of the brain. The brain shrinks and its ability to send communication through a network of neuronal firing is impeded, then eliminated. The cause of this shrinking is a blockage by plaques and tangles that impact and dry up the neuronal channel. We do not know the cause, we do not have a cure (to date). There is no way to permanently delay the diseases progression.

There is no real "formal diagnosis" for Alzheimer's Disease other than an autopsy . However, we know this is not a normal part of aging, and occurs at an average of 1 in 8 people age 65+. If a cure is not discovered, with the massive size of the baby boomer generation, just through their aging over time this disease will turn into epic proportions and financially crush the American healthcare system.

REF: Review these Websites for further information
www.alz.org

Electronic Signals that form memories and thoughts move through an individual nerve cell. These channels are connected by a gap called the *synapse*. When a charge reaches a synapse, it turns into a chemical and travels across the synapse, carrying signals to the other side. They are received at the receptor sites then converted back into an electron pulse whereby the message continues through the neuronal channel up to the next synapse.

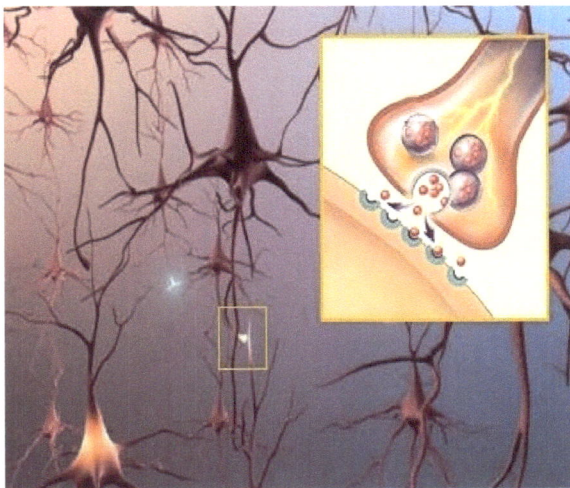

Plaques and tangles (shown in the blue-shaded areas) tend to interfere with the passing of the signal at the receptor site crating a sort of blocking. The neural channel then dries up and dies, not to be regenerated. Because it is permanently gone, the brain has fewer channels to send its thinking commands.

So as the brain shrinks the 8 Thinking skills that run our body become diminished through its blocked inability to send commands.

As a general rule, regarding clinical matters you should not rely solely on the judgement of others or your own observations, use your doctor as a primary information resource. It is suggested that you confer with your doctor on information that you are using to make critical decisions. Start by getting your loved one assessed. So, where to go for an assessment???

Unfortunately, Not every doctor is familiar with the complexities of the dementia assessment process, so you will need to find a doctor who is experienced at diagnosing dementia types. Currently, there is no single test that proves a dementia assessment, although it is possible to achieve 90% accuracy. They use what is called a "clinical Assessment" where through testing all other possible causes are eliminated. This leaves a narrowed list of real possible causes.

NOTE: Everything discussed and reviewed in our books, seminars on our website and in our literature should be considered as a starting point of your understanding. None of what is stated is to be taken as your final piece of information and all information provided should be reviewed with a licensed physician prior to making any decision or taking any action. It is important to always check your information with a licensed professional.

Prior to taking this seminar it is suggested that you have completed an Alzheimer's assessment and have a diagnosis of your loved one. We recommend that you consult with a Brain Institute Team which can be found at the Cleveland Clinic or University Hospital System. Be sure to leave the appointment with a primary diagnosis of your loved one and in which stage of progression is the disease.

We suggest these two groups because they are focused specifically on the brain and understand the assessment process by using a clinical team to perform each assessment.

1. **216.636.5860 Call to set an appointment, Cleveland Clinic Brain Institute Ask for Barbara**

   http://my.clevelandclinic.org/locations_directions/regional-locations/lakewood-hospital/specialties/r.euro.aspx

Get an Assessment: 216-844-2724 Call for appointment, University Hospital Ask for Bonnie.

Or

In other states, contact your local University Hospital System for their Brain Institute Department.

It is recommended that you prepare for the appointment, and not just show up. This is a world that will do more for you if you are prepared and do more for yourself. You can read the Alzheimer's Association website and gain great deal of information that will empower you during the visit. There are test names, lab result information, list of questions to ask, and a check list for what to bring to the appointment. Do these things in preparation of your visit and follow up visits.

It is important that a person who has direct knowledge of the loved ones *"behavior changes and life style"*, be at this appointment.

1. They will provide family history and medication history.
2. During the assessment, an evaluation of the patient will be completed for depression, substance abuse, nutrition, and other conditions that can cause memory loss.
3. A physical exam, blood tests and brain scan will be performed in order to determine what disease is causing the dementia.

Most University Brain Institutes have a team approach that performs these assessments. On their team is a **Neurologist, Pharmacist, Social Worker, Psychologist, Occupational Therapist**. They will each review and profile the patient and then meet as a team to review the case results. This in-depth review is the best way to fully understand the patient's condition. It also creates an important base line and will be used to measure progression in the future.

As a Primary Caregiver: Once you have a diagnosis of Alzheimer's Disease, take the time, now, to find a S*upport Group*. Start early, it is o.k. to shop around and try a few before settling in with the one that is the right fit. This group may be able to help you find a good caregiver and resources to come into your home for daily support.

The first steps include: get a qualified assessment, get a primary diagnosis, understand the current stage, then find a support group. Do not put off finding a support group, they share great advice, and that is what you will need most. Plus they know the pains and problems you will experience and can give insights of what they did in those moments.

ASSIGNMENT: Go on line www.alz.org/cleveland/ or type in your city name. Look up a list of support groups in your area.

18

Keep in mind the initial assessment is a baseline from a list of lab and imaging results. You will be using these tests results as a reference in the future "follow-up" visits with this same clinical team. Once you have a diagnosis, do a google search and a www.youtube search to learn more about that specific disease.

Mini-Cog

The initial test for diagnosing dementia, the mini-cog takes only takes a few minutes to administer and is used as an initial screening for various types of dementia. Most physicians can provide this level of testing. The patient is required to identify three objects in the office, then draw the face of a clock in its entirety from memory, and finally, recall the three items identified earlier. This is a shallow test used to determine if other testing is needed. If failed, then other tests are recommended.

Imaging Tests: CTs, MRIs and Pet Scans (greater detail)

Diagnosing dementia by looking at the structure of the patient's brain by CT or MRI to see if there are any growths, abnormalities or general shrinkage. This raises the accuracy of the diagnosis to 90%. A PET scan administered and reviewed by an expert delivers the most accurate and suggestive results while diagnosing dementia.

Each member of this team will have their own specific diagnostic tools that are used in standardizing the assessment of your loved one. You are paying for these tests and have a right to receive an explanation about each test used, what they measure and what are the final results? These are the questions you should be prepared to ask. Go on the internet and research the test prior to the visit.

Following an assessment, you will be given a diagnosis. Below you will find a list of the most common types of dementia and their causes.

1. Vascular Dementia

This is the second most common form of dementia, caused by poor blood flow to the brain. Often Cardiac conditions, blood clots, or restricted blood flow to the brain.

2. **Mixed Dementia**

   Sometimes dementia is caused by more than one medical condition. This is called mixed dementia. The most common form of mixed dementia is caused by both Alzheimer's Disease and vascular disease.

3. **Dementia with Lewy Bodies (DLB)** this type of dementia is characterized by abnormal protein deposits called Lewy bodies which appear in nerve cells in the brain stem. These deposits disrupt the brain's normal functioning, impairing cognition and behavior and can also cause tremors. DLB is not reversible and has no known cure.

4. **Parkinson's Disease Dementia (PDD)** Parkinson's disease is a chronic, progressive neurological condition, and in its advanced stages, the disease can affect cognitive functioning. Not all people with Parkinson's disease will develop dementia, however. Dementia due to Parkinson's is also a Lewy body dementia. Symptoms include tremors, muscle stiffness and speech problems. Reasoning, memory, speech, and judgment are usually affected. Have your physician identify if PDD is with Lewy Body Dementia.

5. **Frontotemporal Dementia**

   Pick's disease, the most common of the frontotemporal dementia types, is a rare disorder which causes damage to brain cells in the frontal and temporal lobes. Pick's disease affects the individual's personality significantly, usually resulting in a decline in social skills, coupled with emotional apathy.

6. **Mild Cognitive Impairment (MCI)**

   Dementia can be due to medical illness such as HIV/AIDS, medications and a host of other treatable causes. With mild cognitive impairment, an individual will experience memory loss, and sometimes impaired judgment and speech.

The Alzheimer's disease progresses in stages, they are known and identified below. Each stage identifies different levels of brain diminishment. Therefore, declining behaviors are also noticed as the disease progresses. Within each stage a semiannual revisit to the specialist and a re-assessment is completed to determine the progress of the disease. These stages have average timelines, but each person will progress in a declining slope over time, at their own pace.

Stage of Alzheimer's Disease Progression:

1. **Mild -Moderate Cognitive Impairment (MCI)** Stage, 5-7 years duration

2. **Early On-Set Stage** of Alzheimer's disease, 2 years duration

3. **Mild Stage** Alzheimer's disease, 1.5 years duration

4. **Moderate Stage** Alzheimer's disease, 2.5 years

5. **Late Stage** Alzheimer's disease, 2.5 years

6. **End of Life Stage** Alzheimer's disease

Q: What is your loved ones current stage?

NOTES:

_____
_____
_____
_____
_____
_____
_____
_____
_____
_____
_____
_____
_____
_____
_____
_____

Early On-Set Changes in the loved one with Alzheimer's Disease:

In the early on-set stage the person has been experiencing changes in thinking and memory long before it is noticed by others. There can be a decline in judgment and reasoning abilities as well as short term memory loss. Being less able to function in activities and situations can be the end result. Since many daily tasks require decision making and memory skills, with little room for errors the ability to manage money, keep track of multiple bills, or use good judgment when investing and spending money should be of concern.

Changes in language abilities may be evident early in the disease. A change in personality and their ability to reason or think about the needs of others may diminish. It doesn't mean they are selfish, that part of the brain is dying and they can't do this level of thinking anymore. But, it is not as sever in Early On-Set as it will become in the Moderate and Late Stages.

They may deny a problems exist, making excuses or joking. Their anxiety and depression may compound their thinking ability. This may be a good time for them to have counseling from a licensed therapist who can help the person to accept these changes. Also, consider that some of these symptoms may come from their current medications or other conditions in their environment. Always consider medication as a possible cause until it is reviewed by a professional.

This is also a good time for the primary caregivers to seek out a therapist for themselves. One that has experience in family caregiving is preferred.

GAIN AN UNDERSTANDING:

- o The Brain has 8 Thinking Skills
- o Changes in the 8 Thinking Skills
- o Primary Caregiver, What to expect

There are several areas of the brain that run our body. As the disease progresses it will likely affect certain parts before other parts. Keep in mind, the brain is shrinking, once these channels dry up they will not be coming back.

Our Brains have "Thinking Skills", there are Eight of them, get to know what they look like in behavior now, so you can judge how they change in the future.

1. Reasoning Skill

2. Judgement

3. Memory

4. Perception

5. Abstract Thinking

6. Language

7. Organizing

8. Attention

The Eight Thinking Skills are those we use every day. This is how our body works when the commands are sent from the brain.

1. Reasoning Skills:

- A person with Alzheimer's Disease is losing their ability to reason. This happens in Early On-Set stage. Asking them to do something they are not able to perform is not a productive therapy when done by someone who is untrained. However, in the right setting, it can be helpful.

- If they appear to not understand. don't talk louder thinking they will reason better. You cannot use increased volume to address reasoning ability. In fact, increased volume will frighten them and create a great deal of confusion.

- The more reasoning you use the more confused they get. And there will be little success negotiating with them. They are not trying to be difficult, they just can no longer do it. So, change your expectations. They understand better from your tone of voice, facial expression, more than the words you use. Going forward words have :less meaning" as they don't make as much sense. Please treat your response out of an act of love, not frustration or anger.

- Eventually, when it is time to do things, you may have to step in and do it with them. You are not being controlling, it is in an act of love.

2. Judgement Skills:

- Judgement Skill will increasingly become impaired.

- Changes in critical judgement that impact safety, to how they get dressed for the weather.

- You have to gauge this to determine where you step in. Knowing what stage you are in may help.

- You have to think in advance of their decision to determine the result their action will create. Try to be in-front of what they will do next.

3. Memory Skills:

o Short term memory declines, names of items, some family and friend names.

o Difficulty remember complex instructions, directions to places. New thing are likely not going to go well.

o Keeping their dignity is a caring goal. They often know mistakes are made and just can not control how it is done correctly. Be empathic, be understanding, the person inside wants to please you. It's that this dam disease that won't let them.

4. Perception Skills:

o Misinterpreting information is often seen in Alzheimer's Disease.

o Visual: they will see something and interpret it in the wrong way. A dark spot on the floor may be seen as a hole in the ground.

o When looking in the mirror it may be seen as some unknown person attacking them. This may come later in the disease progression.

5. Abstraction Skill:

o This is impeded. Abstract concepts can include the space of time and location. They cannot reconcile the what and when to where.

o Saying we are going to go shopping tomorrow, they might not understand, shopping or tomorrow.

o How to use pill trays, they don't know what the "M" on the box means.

o In the beginning post notes, calendars and pill boxes will work. As it progresses these will not be useful. You need to monitor as to when this happens, then stop using them.

6. Language Skills:

o Structuring the right words for a sentence will become more difficult. Using the wrong words will become more frequent. Do not bother correcting them, accept these parts of the brain are now gone; this is a part of the caregiver journey. Fill in for them to help complete sentences, do so without drawing attention to your help.

o Routines are a good thing. Doing the same thing every day is good for them, they like it. Talk in a way they would talk. Don't use complicated words.

7. Attention Skill:

o They will not be able to stay at a task for long periods of time.

o They will have difficulty in a conversation staying on the topic

In Early On-Set stage the primary caregiver will need to assist with activity reminders at this point in the disease progression. It is preferred that the loved one does as much on their own as they can, given the changes that are taking place. Keep in mind the days of making them remember are over. So try to make simple changes in the environment, in your approach and in your expectations. There is no reason to panic. Slower is their new life rhythm. A more relax less complicated rhythm.

When the family (in Early On-Set stage) reviews the loved ones competency it is often related to critical issues like managing money, business affairs, and driving. If the loved one refuses help, the family can benefit from counseling, to learn coping skills, also the councilor can be a third person who can create the good cop bad cop switch. When the loved one is impulsive or unsafe, primary caregiver must take over the responsibilities of the persons affairs given they can no longer handle it themselves.

In the Moderate stage is when the family members start taking on more of their assigned roles, this will provide a greater relief for the primary caregiver. As family members step up and accept responsibilities a continuity of the same message comes from all those around their loved one. This creates a more stable environment for everyone.

The first big step for the primary caregiver is when the family members accept the changes and the diagnosis. This allows the family members to begin learning about the disease and realizes these changes are not purposeful or vindictive but are the result of the disease process causing impaired thinking. The disease will change over stages, and thus the loved one gradually changes within each stage. There is rarely a leveling off point. Just when you think things are getting normal, the normal changes.

As a main goal of caregiving, things should be kept as normal and usual as possible. Family and friends should use this time while the person can still understand and participate in discussions to make future plans. Use this time to lay the groundwork for what's ahead. The person with Alzheimer's disease will become increasingly dependent on others. Feelings of trust and security are very important to a person who is confused and aware of losing control. To them, their fear and anxiety are very real.

Dignity is the key to being loving. Treat their abilities in a way that keeps their dignity.

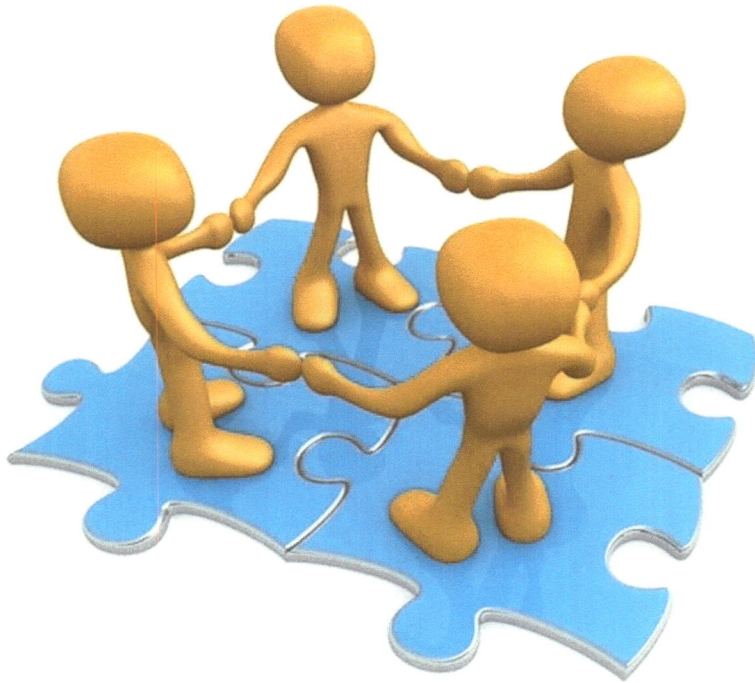

SESSION THREE

Connecting the Progression with its Dementia Behavior

Gain An Understanding:

- o New Characteristics in Behavior, What to expect, Early On-Set Stage
- o Activity Management, In Early On-Set Stage
- o How to support the primary caregiver as a family

An Understanding: The New Characteristic of Behavior, What to Expect

---

1. **Mild decline, a beginning of deficits in thought processes:**

As the disease progresses, taking in information for the loved one becomes more problematic. It will present in areas such as short term memory, their judgment, reasoning, and planning. Minor problems may be noticed in conversation with an inability to complete a thought. The performance of some daily tasks--for example, reading, writing, calculating, managing finances, driving, meal preparation, shopping, or following a medication schedules. Other tasks such as dressing, grooming, and bathing are not done as usual. Be sure to monitor their environment for hazardous activities.

Orientation:

The loved one may become confused when in unfamiliar places. Plan ahead to reduce complicated environments.

Language and Communication:

Only minor problems occur regarding speech in Early On-Set Stage. The changes may include word-finding or forgetting names. They may begin to withdraw from groups due to fear of making errors. Some anger arises from the frustration of being unable to explain themselves when tested or confronted. Try to avoid arguments and confrontational interactions when with others.

Emotional and Behavioral Changes:

You can expect emotional reactions that may be similar to the way they used to cope with problems in the past. Consider their decline in their thinking ability as emotional factors related to the behavior changes. They notice these changes, they read your behavior, they still have feelings and you can share your love or share your frustration. If the later, they will likely not be able to say: "I'm sorry that I am doing this to you".

2. Common Emotional Responses:

Depression is common as a reaction to their awareness of impairment. It starts in the Early On-Set Stage when they are diagnosed as they notice they are changing and can not control it.

Withdrawal from people and situations can be used as a means of protection from their new inabilities.

Anxiety may go up as attempts to carry out usual activities become more difficult.

Agitation, frustration, and anger may erupt at the inability to comprehend, interact and complete tasks.

Denial Sometimes they use humor to redirect the attention off of themselves.

Impulsivity, Because they may not think ahead, this may cause a disruption or danger.

Impaired judgment coupled with agitation and denial often lead to behaviors without thought of consequences.

The more aggressive behavior may present in the latter part of Mild Stage, through Moderate and into Late stages. R~House Alzheimer's Family Learning Center has seminars for each stage of the disease progression. This way you are never alone. We encourage the family sign up for each next stage prior to needing it.

3. The General Guidelines for Care

Consider, in the beginning you can encourage the use of written notes, daily checklists, date books, reminders. But don't stress out when they no longer use them, this is a short lived skill. They are likely not able to learn complex new things. When the person cannot understand issues, anger and agitation often escalate. One will find confusion to be the source of many behavioral issues. You should focus on creating a less confusing environment. You are now an "Environment Specialist", you control their environment.

Watch for signs of frustration and anxiety that may indicate a task is too complicated for the person to understand. Break the task down into more manageable, separate steps and monitor completion of the task. Work together on the task. By beginning to do tasks and activities together, you can give subtle guidance and allow the person to feel a sense of accomplishment. This can turn into quality time for both of you, it's a part of your journey together.

When necessary, take over responsibility for the task without drawing attention to the fact

Suggest jobs that need to be done, for example, yard work or repetitive housework tasks such as vacuuming. Its o.k. to point out safety issues, but monitor them, that role is still yours.

Maintaining social contacts and involvement with others is an important goal for their care during Early On-Set.

Encourage independent involvement in the community. Encourage friends to continue their social contacts. If transportation is an issue (e.g., to and from a daily program), it is advisable to begin using community-based transportation services at this stage. At later stages of thinking impairment, it is more difficult for the person to adapt to changes in routine.

An Understanding: Activity Management in Early On-Set Stage

Independence and Basic Care:

Independent Living is usually possible at the beginning of Early On-Set Stage, however they will progress and you should be planning in advance where the next step will take you. This is especially true if the person has been living alone or in an unfamiliar setting. By contacting your physician an At Home Occupational Therapist can be ordered to complete an assessment of the right level of support required for independent living.

Travel:

Driving issues will be a part of the journey. It is not a matter of "If" more a matter of "When". Ask your physician to address this issue with them. This can avoid the person's anger towards a family member.

 Be prepared for the time when a person can no longer drive, other transportation must be made available to replace this loss. It's not fair to cut them off and leave them with no options. Plan ahead.

Finances and Spending:

Managing finances include keeping track of income, paying bills, writing checks, or doing other banking activities. These often becomes more difficult early in the course of the disease. Family may be unaware of the difficulty with money management until something happens or there is a crisis. Money management activities should be simplified. For example, try setting up auto pay for monthly bills like utilities. With their credit cards you will want to monitor them so these are best left for manual bill paying. Given the disease, this happens in most cases. So prepare for it.

Legal and financial planning is necessary when a family receives a diagnosis of dementia. Early planning will permit the person to have their estate managed in a manner consistent with their wishes. Gather together all legal documents and have them reviewed by a license professional. Also, purchase the book "The Alzheimer's Journey, Its time to get organized" by Roy P. Poillon for a step by step process in getting financial, legal and medical documents organized. www.amazon.com

Shopping involves not only handling money, but also making decisions about what to buy, they have difficulty remembering the items. The Mall can be an overload, with visual, smell, and sound coming at the person on purpose, all at the same time, to influence their buying. It maybe too much for your loved one to process. Try a walk in the park.

Food Preparation and Eating:

Preparing meals may be an activity that a person with early dementia can do, especially if cooking is familiar. But less so with more complex recipes. Cooking with them can be time spent together, bring your patience, sense of humor and plan for everything to take longer.

Medication Management:

Medication management can sometimes be done independently. More often, caregivers are needed to monitor the use of medication trays, or to set them up as in using a pill box with labels. Eventually the pill box will not make sense to them.

Telephone Use:

Phoning abilities tend to change for some at the beginning of Early On-Set. Their ability to have an interesting conversation will decline, remembering things, conversing, and taking a message becomes more difficult.

Work and Leisure:

Volunteer work that involves simple, repetitive tasks can be a productive use of time. But, here too it will have a limited timeline where tasks can be completed to be a value to the organization. Your loved one may become embarrassed and then anxious about others seeing them in this condition. Try to create a balance with this in mind.

Housekeeping, and yard work activities should be monitored for beginning difficulty. Contributing to the family is important for self-esteem. Find tasks that are in line with their ability.

Working together can allow for meaningful experience and quality time together. Find group projects where others can participate. As some activities begin to cause frustration, be prepared with a list of replacement activities. Encourage relatives to initiate outings on a regular basis - restaurants, tours, special events (home and garden shows, sports).

Preferred hobbies and crafts should be continued; new activities will require encouragement, repetition of instructions, and perhaps some demonstration. Some assistance with directions may now be necessary, and less complex versions of favorite crafts may be more successful.

- Cognitive Decline Stages :
    o Ranges from no symptoms (but disease is present) to forgetfulness and loss of object names.
- Early Dementia Stage – the Early On-Set Stage: Duration 5-7 years
    o Difficulty in Concentrating
    o Short term memory loss
    o Trouble Completing complex tasks
    o Denial about symptoms
- Mild Dementia Stage: Duration 2 years
    o Require assistance in getting dressed
    o Trouble remembering names when introduced to new people
    o Having greater difficulty performing tasks in social or work settings
    o Losing or misplacing a valuable object
    o Increasing trouble with planning or organizing
- Moderate Dementia Stage: Duration 2.5 years
    o Requires extensive assistance in daily living tasks.
    o Forgetfulness of events or about one's own personal history, names of close family members
    o Feeling moody or withdrawn, especially in socially or mentally challenging situations
    o Being unable to recall their own address or telephone number or the high school or college from which they graduated
    o Confusion about where they are or what day it is
    o Trouble controlling bladder and bowels in some individuals
    o Changes in sleep patterns, such as sleeping during the day and becoming restless at night
    o An increased risk of wandering and becoming lost
- Late Dementia Stage: Duration 2.5 years
    o Require full-time, around-the-clock assistance with daily personal care
    o Require high levels of assistance with daily activities and personal care
    o The ability to walk, sit and, eventually, swallow
    o Have increasing difficulty communicating
    o Become vulnerable to infections, especially pneumonia
- End of Life Alzheimer's Disease: Support the person to live as well as possible: Comfort Care.

    o Including pain relief and management of other symptoms
    o Require assistance in toileting, eating, moving from bed to chair.
    o their spiritual beliefs and needs.
    o Kept comfortable and free from distressing symptoms
    o Surrounded by those close to them to give love and compassion.

Palliative care professionals at a local hospice specialist from a team of professionals can give personal advice on the options available at this stage. We suggest you not assume you know all that is offered, as some provide different programs. The person should always have an up-to-date care plan that includes end of life plans and is shared with those involved in the person's care. Some areas have special staff who co-ordinate end of life care for people with dementia. Ask the GP, community nurse or local hospice (if you have one) about what is available n your area.

If they are getting something wrong,
do not bother with correcting them. Let it go.

The Connection: Disease Progresses, Behavior Changes, Family Gets Educated-United-Organized.

First Step: Get Educated, The Alzheimer's Journey, Connecting the Puzzle Pieces (Seminar)

Second Step: Get United, 7 Dynamics in an Alzheimer's Family (Seminar)

Seminar One: An Understanding, Gain knowledge about the assessment process, disease and how to make decisions as a family. Agree to a common core of family values.

Seminar Two: An Empowerment, Use the knowledge to move into critical issues in each stage of the disease, use the families spiritual faith practices.

Seminar Three: A Proactive Plan, Distribute the responsibilities and work load into assigned roles, then make a plan of action at the beginning of each stage.

Third Step: Get Organized, The Alzheimer's Journey, It's time to Get Organized (Seminar)

Use the "Personal Attaché" product found in the book, The Alzheimer's Journey, It's Time To Get Organized. Order Here: www.amazon.com search Roy Poillon all books will come up.

Setting-up Role & Responsibilities Sharing

Financial Estate: consolidate all the financial assets together into "The Financial Attaché Binder"

Legal Documents: consolidate all the legal documents together into "The Legal Attaché Binder",

Medical Records: consolidate all the Medical Records and Health Profile together into a portable, "The Medical Attaché Binder"

In Home Safety Environment done by an Occupational Therapist, ordered by your doctor

Support Network: create a list of community support to include businesses, non for profit agencies and government agencies. Place it in a binder, "The Support Network Binder".

Spiritual Faith Network: create a list of church contacts that offer ministries and services from the church in areas for the family to utilize at home or in a facility. Place these services and contacts in a binder, "The Spiritual Faith Network Binder".

All these seminar books can be found on www.amazon.com search Roy Poillon

Accessing the 4 Primary Support Structure:
1. **The Family Support Structure:** The family members are their own resource support structure for the primary caregiver and loved one.
2. **The Church Support Structure:** The church is a resource support structure for the family members, primary caregiver and loved one.
3. **The Community Support Structure:** The community (professional services, medical, govt agencies and non for profits) is a support structure for the family members, primary caregiver and loved one.
4. **The Employer Support Structure:** The employer is a support structure for the primary caregiver.

Also, learn how are the 7 Dynamics in an Alzheimer's Family model in each stage.

Use The 7 Dynamics in an Alzheimer's Family Model:
1. Families Core Values
2. The disease, how it progresses
3. Family Decisions Making Model
4. Facing The Critical Issues
5. Managing Dementia Related Behavior
6. Spiritual Faith Practices
7. Roles and Responsibilities

Each stage requires a separate seminar for learning. This is because different critical issues take place as the disease progress. Likewise, new or more pronounced behaviors are presented.

Take These Three Seminars

To strengthen the Family Support Structure, take these three seminars.

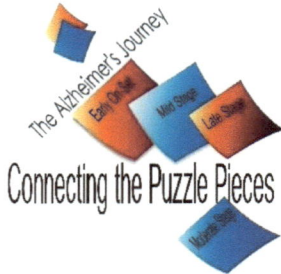

The Alzheimer's Journey, Connecting the Puzzle Pieces, each stage of the disease progression brings about new critical issues, decisions and requirements for proactive planning. The "Connecting the Puzzle Pieces is a five-book series, one for each stage, with a seminar on what to do in each stage. Stages: Early On-Set Stage, Mild Stage, Moderate Stage, Late Stage, End of Life Stage. One Seminar for each stage.

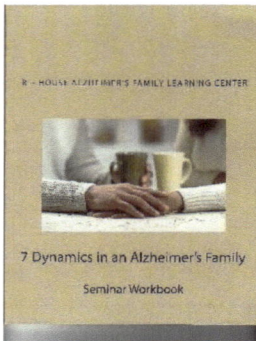

The 7 Dynamics in an Alzheimer's Family, unites the family around the primary caregiver and loved one. There is a lot of work to do as a family. This seminar outlines where to get started. In the seminar the attendees learn how to unite the family, get an understanding of the disease, and how it progresses. They learn how to manage dementia related behavior, create role assignments for family members, and provided templates for creating a proactive plan. Three Seminars

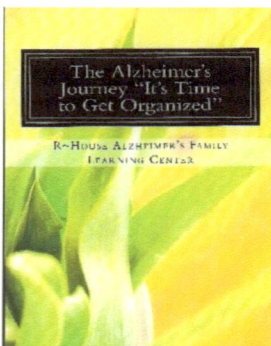

The Alzheimer's Journey, It's Time to get Organized, getting the family organized in the Alzheimer's journey is a matter of taking the right steps. These steps are outlined and reviewed in this seminar. The workbook outlines what to organize, provides templates for setting up organizing binders, planning templates and reference resources. Getting organized reduces stress, save money and gives the family a position of empowerment. Two Seminars

When Alzheimer's Disease is first diagnosed each member of the family will have their world turned upside down.

As they consider all that is in front of them for the next five to twelve years, based on what little they understand about this disease, the future will seem dark and daunting. This is perfectly understandable.

The problem exist that neither their acute care hospital, the physician office or their HMO will take the time to help them learn what is needed to navigate the Alzheimer's Disease journey.

This is a time when the person must pick up the pieces themselves, get united as a family, get organized and get educated on each stage of the disease. R~House Alzheimer's Family Learning Center has gather part of the information required to move forward with their lives into this journey. Their experience will become one of learning, gathering, problem solving and loving.

There is good news; they do not have to travel this journey alone, we provide learning materials for each stage. In fact, from a formation of their spiritual faith and trust in God, no one is ever alone.

The Foundation: For most families the foundation of who they truly are as a family, are found inside their core family values. These core values become a compass or guide point that helps to keep them on the right path. The core values are used to help make critical decisions, sustain through intense arguments between family members and gives confidence to move forward when all the alternatives are unacceptable. Knowing your family core values, "matters". Also, knowing your core spiritual faith practices, "matters". Plan to use both.

The connection between progression and behavior is from the brain shrinking, neuronal cells and channels are dying and this limits the 8 Thinking skills to send commends which impacts the loved ones behavior. This is important to know. But, it is equally important is to understand that these things happen over time, not all at once. Once you see a certain thinking skill start to diminish you can expect that decline to continue. It does not turn itself around and get better later.

For this reason there are five progressive stages of Alzheimer's and the behavior that occurs. It will typically start in one stage but continue to worsen into and through the following stage.

This is why it is important to identify and learn about what behavior you can expect in each stage. Unfortunately, this is not black and white, where it is certain that a behavior will occur in a specific stage. However, in the law of averages you can paint with a broad brush that it will likely fall somewhere in that area or stage.

For example, we typically do not see hallucinations in Early On-Set stage (except for some Parkinson's Cases), but we do see "Sundowning" , Wandering and Shadowing. So, lets prepare for these behaviors, learn about what skills are needed and what others feel is the best way to respond. After all, you kind of know that it is coming, so get organized and get ready.

Because nothing will remain the same, overtime there will be a lot of decisions required of the family. The critical issues that will arise in each stage can be taxing when you do not see them coming and have no plan on what resource structure to use.

Decision making and critical issues are something that a family can come together to make the journey more successful and less stressed.

~ Seminar Break ~

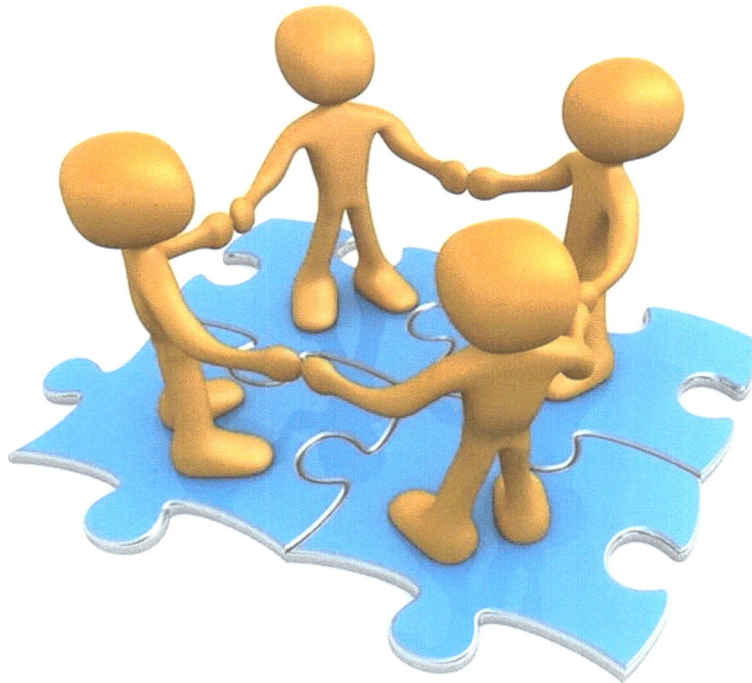

SESSION FOUR

Connecting the Decision Making Model

to Critical Issues

I.   3rd Dynamic Decision Making Model

II.   4th Dynamic Facing Critical Issues in Alzheimer's Disease

Please watch the link video prior to the meeting.

https://www.youtube.com/watch?v=kpInfNUp6Ak

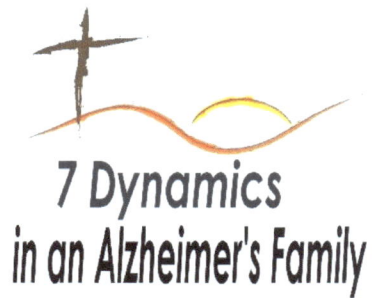

7 Dynamics
in an Alzheimer's Family

3rd Dynamic

The Decision Making Model

Grieving and Decision Making

In the progression of the disease, a great deal of decision making will be required of the family. Each member will likely be at a different level of accepting the disease, which will likely impact their ability to make demanding complex decision. For this reason a standard model for decision making will be a helpful family tool.

The Dynamic of Decision Making includes Anticipatory grief

From Wikipedia, the free encyclopedia

The five stages (denial, anger, depression, bargaining and acceptance) proposed by Elisabeth Kübler-Ross in her model of grief to describe the process by which people cope after a loss can also be present in anticipatory grief. Anxiety, dread, guilt, helplessness, hopelessness, and feeling overwhelmed are also common. However, it is important to note that anticipatory grief is not simply normal grief begun earlier.[1]

Features identified specifically with anticipatory grief include heightened concern for the declining person, rehearsal of the death and attempts to adjust to the consequences of the death. The period can allow people to resolve issues with the declining person and to say goodbye.[1] It may provide some sense of orientation and access to the grieving process. For some, it prompts conscious closure before the end/loss.[2]

Grief happening prior to a loss presents a compounding issue of isolation because of a lack of social acceptance. Anticipatory grief doesn't usually take the place of post-loss grief: there is not a fixed amount of grief to be experienced, so grief experienced before the loss does not necessarily reduce grief after the death.[1] However, there may be little grieving after the loss due to anticipatory grief.[3]

How often anticipatory grief occurs is a subject of some controversy. For example, a study of widows found that they stayed with their husbands until the death and could only mourn once the death had occurred. Researchers suggest that to start to grieve as though the loss has already happened can leave the bereaved feeling guilt for partially abandoning the patient.[1]

42

During the progression of the illness, the security and protectiveness of the caregiver also increases. Bouchal, Rallison and Sinclair discuss that, "the strong need to offer protection was part of the anticipatory mourning experience of striving to be with in the present" (2015).

In the process of anticipatory grief, family members also begin to prepare and reflect on how their lives will be once their loved one passes. There are many ways in which to perform reflection. These ways include: "...reading, journaling, thinking, and reflecting about how life might be like without their partner." The journal also expands on the premise that the preparation process is not an individual process. Those who are affected by the impending death often look towards one another for support as well as others who are involved in care such as nurses and social workers (Bouchal et al., 2015).

A direct correlation exists between anticipatory grieving and the caregiver's quality of life. In a quantitative study conducted by Al-Gamal and Long, the effect of a pediatric cancer diagnosis on parents had a negative impact on the majority of study participants. More specifically, parents reported experiencing increasing stress and a decrease in physical and mental health – all of which affect the process of anticipatory grief (2010).

Ultimately, anticipatory grieving is an extremely dynamic process that differs between individuals. The outcomes of the grieving process depend on the preparation of death and the anticipatory grief process. In making decisions we have to take into account our current situation, from the state of mind where we are being asked to make a decision. After all we are in grieving, and yet expected to think with complete clarity. We may or may not be impacted by our grieving process, but if it is impacted by grieving, we would be well advise to take this into consideration. Therefore, knowing what phase of grieving we are, as a part of the grieving process might be helpful before we begin the decision-making process.

EXAMPLE: if we are in the fourth stage of the grieving process, then we are "negotiating" with the acceptance of the dying process. This being our mental state may influence how we make a decisions. We may be more inclined to *negotiate* in our decision-making. This is why a standard model is important to use. It forces out the emotions and outside influences of our world, in order that we make value based, fact informed, logical decisions. Given that there are five stages to grieving, then we will not want these five different stages to transcend and negatively impact the years over which a number of critical decisions will be made for the care of our loved one. This is why R~House Alzheimer's Family Learning Center is recommending a standard decision-making model.

Kübler-Ross Grief Cycle

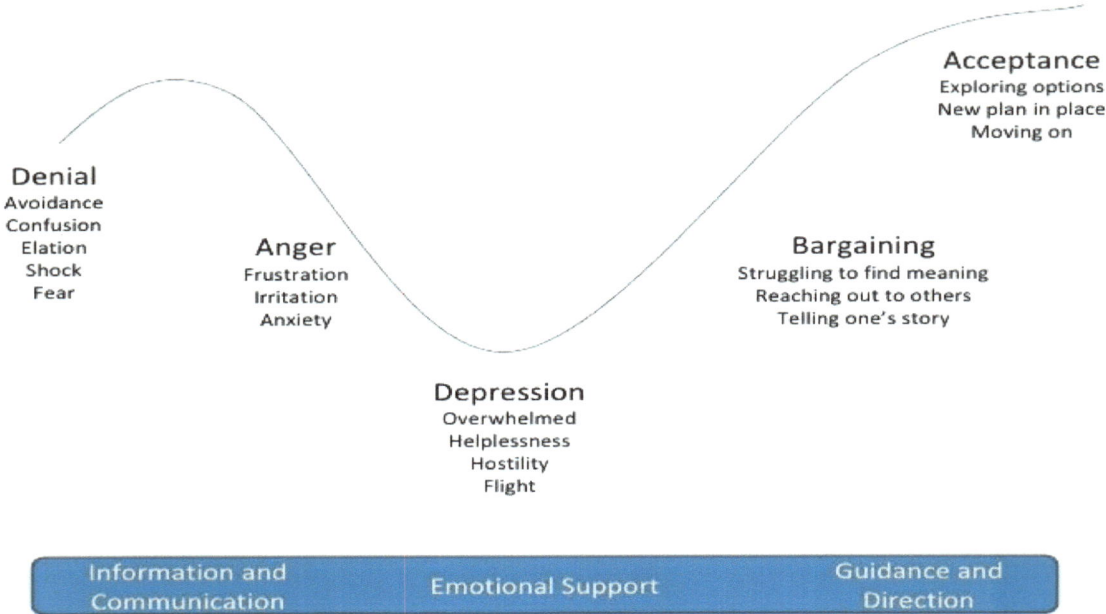

Denial
Avoidance
Confusion
Elation
Shock
Fear

Anger
Frustration
Irritation
Anxiety

Depression
Overwhelmed
Helplessness
Hostility
Flight

Bargaining
Struggling to find meaning
Reaching out to others
Telling one's story

Acceptance
Exploring options
New plan in place
Moving on

Information and Communication	Emotional Support	Guidance and Direction

Because each member of the family will be in a different phase of the grieving process, collaborating for a combined decision will be even more difficult. Using a standard decision making model can help to normalize each persons participation, so alike characteristics are considered without having to weight some over others.

USING THE DECISION MAKING MODEL

PURPOSE: The purpose of a family meeting is multi-faceted. It can serve to communicate information regarding the loved one's situation, or the status of family members. The meeting can also be used to *make critical decisions* or to determine role responsibilities. In many cases it is all of these.

TASK: In order to make effective decisions as a group, an agreed upon process is important to ensure participation and success in making the best decision. As a family, you are tasked to *make many decisions* in the Alzheimer's journey. This model will provide a frame work that when used will be helpful to gain the best insight to the problem, a criteria of importance, to consider the options and weigh the possible outcomes.

CONDITION: By gathering as a group to learn about the Alzheimer's disease, the family has taken the first step in making strong decisions. The second step is to understand the stages and what behavior will occur in each stage. In the final step by gathering as a family, review the family values, understand how to use a "Family Decision Model", Assigning Roles and Responsibilities. Then set a strategy for the next few months. This is a great process to follow and is the right place for the family to get started.

STANDARD: The standard is that <u>each person will participate</u>. The individual family member will take on an assigned role and be responsible to achieve the assignments in that role to their best ability. They will seek assistance when needed and approach all areas of the family, with respect, dignity and a positive, "Can Do" attitude

The Decision Making Model:

First: Identify exactly what happened

Second: Analyze the situation, what caused this to happen

Third: Gather information

Fourth: Create a Criteria for a best solution

Fifth: Choose the best solution

Sixth: Who needs to be involved in the solution

To follow are decision making exercises. Take the time to practice or choose a topic your family is currently dealing with and apply the model.

First Step: Identify Exactly What Happened

Exercise *: What Happened?*
Identify the details of the situation? (what happened, How did it happen, Who was involved?)

What:_____
_____
_____How:_____
_____
_____
_____Who:_____
_____
_____

Identify what you would have like to have happened?

_____
_____
_____
_____
_____
_____
_____
_____
_____
_____
_____
_____

Second Step: Analyzing the Situation

Every problem has a situation that surrounds it, <u>and inside the situation typically is where you will find the solution</u> to the problem. By analyzing the situation more closely, the solution will typically present itself. It will then be clarified and used in your decision making process.

Exercise :We will take a look at the problem that impacts the situation. (what went wrong)

1 Assessing the Problem: (Describe exactly what is happening that is not working?)

_____

_____

_____

_____

_____

_____

_____

2 Identify, what is causing this to happen?

_____

_____

_____

3 In what areas did this create an impacting or disruption?

_____

_____

_____

_____

_____

4 What is the number one contributing factor?

_____

_____

_____

_____

Third Step: Gathering Information

It may seem unnecessary to have a segment that reviews "Gathering Information" however, this is a critical part of the decision making process and can significantly impact the quality of your decision and its outcome.

There are three types of information gathering sources to consider:

1. The Primary Source information, The person it happened to, or who was there when it happened?
2. The Secondary Source information, He Said - She Said.
3. The Gut Feeling Source, no one person saw it happen, but I think this is what occurred.

All of the above information types are reasonable to include in the decision making model.

The Primary Source: Prepare a list of questions and then go to the primary source for answers. At times you may not know which is the best questions to ask. So research the questions, then go ask them.

Example: If you are considering "moving your loved one into a facility" (critical issue), go to the facility and take a tour. Do not just read their website, listen to someone else's opinion about the facility or telephone them for a few answers. You will need to go directly to them as they are the "primary source" of information. You should come with a prepared list of questions in order to have an accurate understanding of their facility. Search the internet for questions to ask.

The Secondary Source: This is a good resource to consider using when making a decision. The Secondary source is valuable because it allows others to provide information about your search for answers. From Secondary Sources you may find other topics or questions that need to be considered.

There are two areas that you need to be aware of; 1. The source of the secondary information. Who are they, what authority do they speak from, why are they providing this information. 2. Is this information a direct correlation to the topic that you are researching. Be careful, sometimes in secondary search it becomes tempting to seek out information that proves your premises to be correct. That is called bias. We want to avoid being bias, just the facts please!

The Gut Feeling: This is a combination of your past experiences, your family upbringing, your spiritualty, and your cultural values and beliefs. They are all wrapped into one feeling of an emotional response. It should not be ignored and rarely should it be the only information feedback that is used in making an informed "Value Based Decision".

Identifying Reasonable Options

The process of identifying reasonable options can only come after you understand the problem, considered your values, reviewed some of the considerations and circumstances as you continue to gather more information.

Once you complete the information gathering phase of decision making process, it is important to know when to eliminate ideas that are not a good fit, consider only those ideas that will work best. Use your values when considering options, use prayer for guidance, let the Holy Spirit take charge and follow what you believe God would have you do.

Exercise: What are the top three pieces of gathered information?

INFORMATION GATHERING CARD

Gathered Information:

_____

_____

_____

_____

_____

_____

_____

_____

_____

_____

Fourth Step: Criteria for Solution

Exercise: Does your solution qualify for consideration?

CRITICAL CRITERIA, *final Review*

1. Will this action ensure safety for your loved one? ___T ___F
2. Do you have the resources needed to complete these tasks? ___T ___F
3. Is your time table realistic? ___T ___F
4. Do you understand the negative impact(s) your actions may create? ___T ___F
5. Is this an action something that you would want others to take on your behalf? ___T ___F

Set up your own critical criteria as a filter to ensure the best decisions are made. Remember to review your decisions with your clinical team.

Fifth Step: Choose the Best Solution

Exercise: Take your decision and place it here:

_____

We will do the following:

_____
_____
_____
_____
_____
_____
_____
_____
_____
_____
_____

Our expected outcome is:

_____
_____
_____
_____
_____
_____
_____
_____
_____
_____
_____

Sixth Step: Share who needs to be involved in this solution

Name: _____ Phone: _____ Email Address: _____

1.

2.

3.

4.

5.

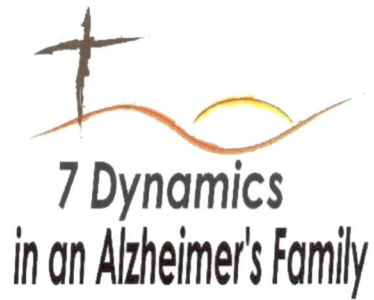

**7 Dynamics
in an Alzheimer's Family**

4th   Dynamic

Facing Critical Issues

CRITICAL ISSUES

1. Getting an assessment and semi-annual follow up assessments

2. Learning about the disease

3. Forming a unified family

4. Understanding the disease behavior

5. Driving and setting up alternatives

6. Building a support network

7. Developing spiritual faith practices around the Alzheimer's journey

8. Assigning roles and responsibilities

9. Placement into a facility

10. Responding to issues at the facility

11. Getting educated about the End of Life journey

12. Preparing for probate

You can add your own to this list.

Exercise # 1: *(Getting an Assessment and semi-annual follow up assessments)*

From Roles and Responsibilities in an Alzheimer's Family workbook.

What will each member of the family do in order to complete this task

1. Learn about the Assessment process and inform the family

2. Organize the medical records binder

3. Coordinate a post assessment family meeting

4. Address other critical issues that come up from the assessment and re-assessments

Prioritize venues that will meet the family's needs.

1. On Line Education

2. Seminar Training

3. Key Websites

4. Selected www.Youtube.com channels

5. Published books on key topics of the disease and caregiving

---

Exercise # 3: *(Forming a Family Meeting)*

All members should attend these meeting in person or by Skype/conference call.

1. Create an agenda to send out prior to the meeting

2. Request assignments to present by other members at the meeting

3. Take notes on key issues discussed and distribute after the meeting

4. State clearly what each person will be doing after the meeting

5. Set a date, time and location for the next meeting

This is more than just learning about what the behavior will look like. The real understanding comes from knowing how to manage the behavior.

- Shadowing

- Sun downing

- Repetitive Calling

- Repetitive Talking

- Aggressive Behavior

- Grooming/Bathroom

- Incontinence

- Hallucinations

- Pain

Notes:

The best advice is to have your primary care physician handle this. You have him write a prescription that reads: NO MORE DRIVING. On his prescription pad. That way later when it is being debated, you can pull it out and use it.

Other resources is to have a "behind the wheel" test done at the DMV.

The spark plug wire can be removed and you would tell them that the car is broken. Take it away and keep

telling them that it is at the garage, parts are being ordered and it should take several weeks.

Notes:

In the development of a Support Network, the idea is to include those areas of support that you will need both now and in the future.

- Medicare Advisor: Tami Glover

- My New Villa: Jill

- Assessment: Cleveland Clinic and University Hospital Systems Brain Institutes

- On Line Training: Healthcare Interavctive.com

- Home Health Aid Companies: Senior Helpers, Home Instead, Visiting Angles

- Financial Advisors: W.A. Smith

- Eldercare Attorney's: Rachael Kalb

- Realtor: Jeff Brandon, Russe l Realty

- Family Counseling

- Disposable Medical Supplies: www.sheildhealthcare.com , www.byramhealthcare.com Incontinence

  supplies, wound and skin ca e

- Medical Equipment: Apria Healthcare

- Home Healthcare and Hospice: Western Reserve Hospice, Heartland Home Healthcare and Hospice,

  VNA.

These are a few examples, search by category, find three and interview them about their services. Do this before you need to use them.

Notes:

Exercise #7: Developing spiritual faith practices around the Alzheimer's journey

In the Early On-Set stage you will have more time to complete a Spiritual Retreat than the time you will have

later in the disease. We recommend subscribing to an on line site, www.formed.org and begin with "30 Days to

Morning Glory" a self guided spiritual retreat for consecrating yourself to Jesus Christ through the Blessed

Mother. You will relearn a great deal about the practice of your Catholic faith in this retreat.

Notes:

The Roles & Responsibilities exercise is contained in a separate document. However, it is a part of the family's critical issues. The importance of the family working together cannot be stressed enough. It has emotional, health and spiritual implications and cannot be ignored.

By gathering as a family to make decisions, by learning at seminars together and praying with each other, your family can experience an enriched journey in this phase of your family's life.

Notes:

Exercise #9: Placement into a facility

- This is a complex point and requires time and diligence if it is to be done in a respectful and responsible manner.

- Plan that you may have to use a difference facility in the future. Therefore, have more than one in mind.

- For this reason I strongly recommend that you hire a Placement Advisor. They understand the process.

- But, you will still need to gather information, get your affairs organized, have multiple meetings and pray as a family. It is a combination of steps and efforts made that will culminate into a quality decision.

Notes:

There are going to be problems at the facility. Some will be due to errors by staff, some by your loved one and some by your misunderstanding of the facts. You can expect all of these and probably some that are not mentioned here.

It is important to visit regularly, at different times of the day and on different days of the week. This will allow you to have an understanding of the shift that is one duty throughout the day, activities and challenges that they are facing with your loved one.

Get to know the Director of nursing.

Meet the Facility Medical Director, every facility has a medical director

Always have a list of questions that are written down so you can leave behind and they can get back with you in a future visit.

Confirm that family members have access to medical records, HIPPA Release Form.

Do your research on the web regarding how to best manage your relationship with the facility care team and management.

Notes:

The End of Life phase of the Alzheimer's journey is similar to other types of End of Life experiences. If there are no other causes of dying, then some of the medical conditions that the loved one will experience are somewhat predictable and can be researched on the internet.

The decision to "know" in advance is yours alone to make. However, certain orders and instructions are recommended to be determined in advance.

1. The loved ones Living Will needs to be in place prior to them diminishing in thought beyond their ability to determine how they want to be treated. This can be set up through a legal document.

2. A DNR "Do Not Resuscitate" is an order/instruction that needs to be clearly explained. Have someone with depth of knowledge in this area review how this is executed.

3. Physician Standing Orders, you will want to know as these change, during the time it is being determined.

Notes:

A separate documents has been provided to your family assigned "executor" . This is a discussion that the family will have in private with the Executor on how he/she understands their role and responsibilities as Executor.

Notes:

Using the 7 Dynamics in an Alzheimer's family model, gives the family a greater resource by including all of the family. It more formally unites the family to work together as one, for one purpose in support of two people (the primary caregiver and the loved one).

Because the model is standardize, each person will contribute in the same way making it easier to combine everyone's input.

Learning the critical issues allow the family time to anticipate the next level of issues that are likely to present. In doing this, better planning, less stress, cost savings and higher quality of care can take place.

However, here again, the family members need to be willing to cooperate and participate in an effort to alleviate the pressure that are on the families primary caregiver.

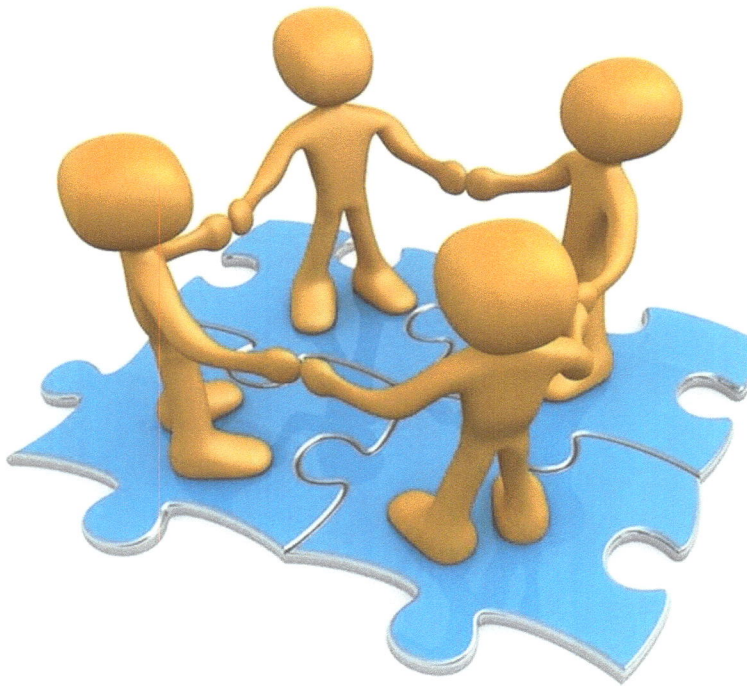

SESSION FIVE

Connecting the Behavior with the 8 Thinking Skills

SECTIONS:

7 Dynamics
in an Alzheimer's Family

5th Dynamic

Managing Dementia Related Behavior

Managing Dementia Related Behavior

The Disease Progresses in 7 Stages (review, go through each)

1. Mild Cognitive Impairment (MCI)
2. Moderate Cognitive Impairment (MCI)
3. Early On Set of Alzheimer's Disease
4. Mild Dementia
5. Moderate Dementia
6. Late Stage Dementia
7. Sever Stage Dementia

Shrinkage Impacts the 8 Thinking Skills (review, go through each)

1. Memory
2. Abstraction
3. Language
4. Attention
5. Perception
6. Reasoning
7. Judgement
8. Motor Skills

Challenges of Aids for Daily Living. (review, go through each) changes by each stage

Bathing
   ☐ Getting into the bath is a challenge
Eating
   ☐ Their ability to sequence the steps in eating
   ☐ Loss of appetite
   ☐ Dental pain, stomach pain, UTI pain
Sleeping
Incontinence is a very big challenge

Ways to manage Dementia Related Behavior

   Understanding their new communication channel: Behavior is their new language to talk and now it will be yours.
   The primary dementia related behavior: (Hitting, Swearing, Spitting, Yelling, wandering, Sun downing). Learn how to assess it, how to respond effectively, how to anticipate it.
   The C.A.R.E.S. approach will make it a lot easier
   Taking control of your loved ones environment
   Key Success "Tools in Reading Their Body Language"

C.A.R.E.S. Model as a Tool

C. connect.

A. Assess the situation before acting.

R. Respond using your assessment.

E. Evaluate the outcome, did it work Why, did it not work Why.

S. Share you experience so others can benefit, repeat what worked avoid what did not work. Always share so it gets passed down the line.

Practical Exercise C.A.R.E.S. Model as a tool

Practice the Approach, slow, low, eye level, forearm and shoulder

Practice the Hand Under Hand brushing teeth, assisting

Practice the Hand Over Hand Soup Spoon, guiding

Other Behaviors, (review Redirecting Skill, go through each)

Repetitive Talking

Shadowing

Sun Downing

Aggressive Behavior

Hallucinations

Skills to use

Hand over Hand

Hand Under Hand

Use a Safety Belt

Pain, Always look for it

It is real, they feel it and can not directly communicate it to you.

Their behavior is often related to pain of some type

Always, consider first pain as a possible reason for aggressive behavior

Find the area, then consult with your doctor to address it

When moving them around pain can be an issue, look for it

Few things will be under the families control. Without training and education, even more will seem uncontrollable, when actually there are some things that can be done. That is why taking learning seminars by stage is a valuable resources. The family should seek to learn what they need for "right now" and look into what they will need to learn in the next stage. There is less value in concern or focusing on what will take place several years down the road. This journey has its path, the path is relatively know and many areas can be identified so the family can be aware and hopefully prepared. As a part of the families learning, Early On-Set Stage is the introduction stage. Other stages will be shorter and have direct application to just that stages issues.

Understanding the Behavior by its name

Using the Tools:

- C.A.R.E.S., redirect, validation

Using Types of Ques and Skills

- Verbal
- Visual
- Touch (tactic) hand under hand, hand over hand

Always look for Pain, Where it hurts, how much does it hurt

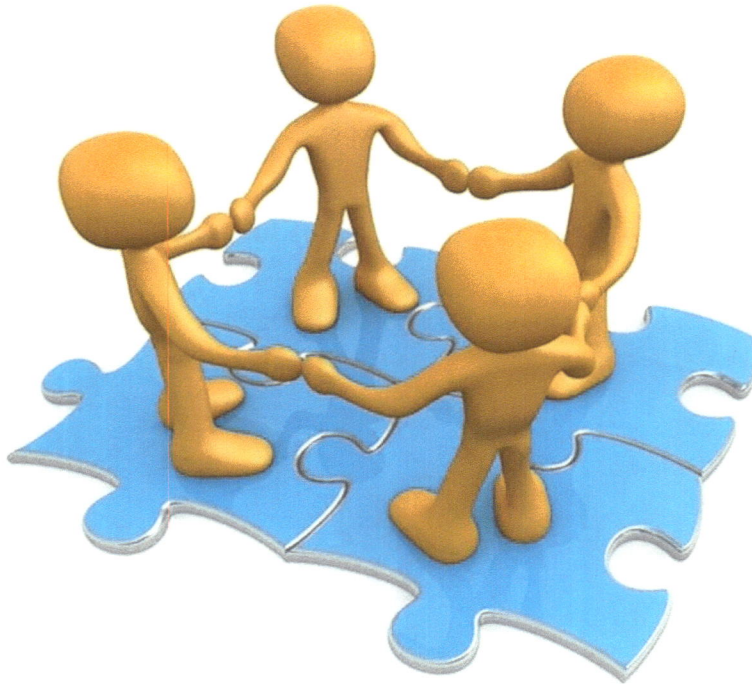

SESSION SIX

Connecting the Journey with its Spirituality

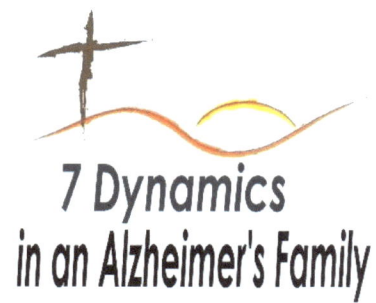

7 Dynamics
in an Alzheimer's Family

6th Dynamic

Spiritual Faith Practices

God teaches us to meet the ones we Love where they are, regardless of their condition.

1 John 4:7-8

Beloved, let us love one another, for love is from God, and whoever loves has been born of God and knows God. Anyone who does not love does not know God, because God is love.

Colossians 3:12-15

Put on then, as God's chosen ones, holy and beloved, compassionate hearts, kindness, humility, meekness, and patience, bearing with one another and, if one has a complaint against another, forgiving each other; as the Lord has forgiven you, so you also must forgive. And above all these put on love, which binds everything together in perfect harmony. And let the peace of Christ rule in your hearts, to which indeed you were called in one body. And be thankful.

In this seminar is a breakdown of the Roles and Responsibilities, the Roles and Responsibilities Plan of Action and how to create a family strategy. This is the seminar where all the past learning, models and skills training come together into a final family plan to unite and work towards the common goal of caring for your loved one with Alzheimer's disease.

Finding answers to what is happening is a major part of the Alzheimer's journey. We search for answers where there may be none. In their place we develop solutions to address what we are dealing with in the moment. Dealing with Alzheimer's is mostly about "what is in the moment". This is when we come to them and meet them where they are, not where we want them to be.

The Soul: In Alzheimer's Disease the soul is not impacted by their inability to communicate as their thinking skills are diminished. If this were the case, then we would have to feel the same about an infant in our arms. In fact, for our loved one this is their last effort to use their spiritual self in sharing their final life expressions. It is from the remainder of who they are, that their more pure sense of self is expressed. They are freed from the entrapments of life's morae's, without inhibitions derived from a pace of self and ego. If you could separate this person from their Alzheimer's disease, what you will find is Love. The same love that God gives to each of our souls, and in them as in us, the soul never dies. The present (now) is part of their eternity as it is, now, also part of ours.

They are vulnerable, deserving of our care and respect. They look to those that love them to tell their story, the stories of themselves (who they are), which they can no longer speak to tell. We hold the identity of "their self" as faithful stewards, to meet them in their new reality, the self that is surrounded by disease and dementia. But, in a much greater way, they are also surrounded by God's love, in His protection according to His plan, with the graces of the Blessed Mother and intercessory prayers of the Saints. The whole being of God surrounds "who they are". They are <u>our loved ones and we are their faithful stewards</u>. Just as it was in the beginning as an infant, it is now and with God will forever be.

The Divine Will: God's Will for us is to love Him and to share in His Divine love. He seeks to be close with all of us, especially those who are sick and suffering. He desires for us to seek Him and His comfort. In this hour of need we should not be distorted by a false understanding of His Divine Will that God punishes as justice for our sins. REF: Jeramiah 29: 11-14. His plan will always be fulfilled together with Him, either now or in some other part of our eternal journey. He knew us before we were born and will be with us, always. So is the Alzheimer's journey, being there with our "loved one" is being closer to Him, as we journey in these final years, in their journey using our combined faith. The faith we have in God and His merciful love. We need to completely trust in Him.

In this three part seminar we will learn about both journeys, the one with Alzheimer's disease and the Spiritual Pathway in Alzheimer's. This is a journey which each member of the family will likely take.

It is stated by many, that in the Alzheimer's journey we come closer to God from our suffering. We find Him there as He has promised. We learn by our faith, to *"Trust in Him"* as He gives to each of us His Divine Mercy.

First Assignment, (Google On-Line): Saint John Paul II Dives In Misericordia

http://w2.vatican.va/content/john-paul-ii/en/encyclicals/documents/

In the care of your loved one, given the worsening of their condition and greater difficulty in their behavior we may find ourselves using a different focus of faith practice in different parts of the journey.

In Early On-Set stage the diagnosis is frightening, it is the unknown of what life will be like moving forward. It is for this reason that we look for knowledge, to answer questions and resolve what is unknown. What we seek from the Lord is WISDOM.

The same is true as the disease progresses and our loved one moves into Mild Stage Alzheimer's. Here we are starting to see the behavior that before was only described as something likely to happen, but now we see it is happening. Here we look to COURAGE from our faith practices.

In the Moderate Stage the condition worsens and behavior is more extreme. We tend to question our commitment, our resolve, our unanswered doubt of fairness. For this we seek a stronger FAITH that God's will is being done and we need to have faith that he is there in these moments.

In the Late Stage of Alzheimer's the decline is appearing to look more like incapacity and it is troubling. For these days we seek HOPE, that it will one day conclude inside his glorious promise of taking our loved ones hand and leading them home.

In End of Life Stage, we see the final months and the ability to accept what is the fait of all; here we use LOVE. Our love for them, God's love for all his children. In Love we find the ability to let go and let God.

STAGE: **FATIH FOCUS:**

EARLY ON-SET STAGE................. Wisdom

MILD STAGE .... Courage

MODERATE STAGE...................... Faith

LATE STAGE .... Hope

END OF LIFE STAGE................ .... Love

In daily practice use the teachings from:

- Scripture
- Saints
- Psalms

For inspiration and meditative prayer.

Early On-Set Stage, Wisdom; what do the scriptures tell us about using wisdom, which saint's provided teachings and what Psalm/Proverbs focused on wisdom. These would be your search fields, reading. In Early On-Set stage ask God for Wisdom.

The assignment page provides some places to get started. You can also ask your deacon, priest, spiritual advisor.

Assignment

View a Video:

Go to www.youtube.com, look up:

Early Onset Alzheimer's disease: Jim's Story | OnMemory.ca

https://www.youtube.com/watch?v=jCoC5IInL88

Read an Article:

www.Alz.org Upper right corner of page is the search box:

Type in: 2015 Alzheimer's Disease Facts and Figures

Visit a Website:

Go to www.Alz.org Upper right corner of page in the search box:

Type in: 10 signs of Alzheimer's

Type in: Check List for Doctor Visit

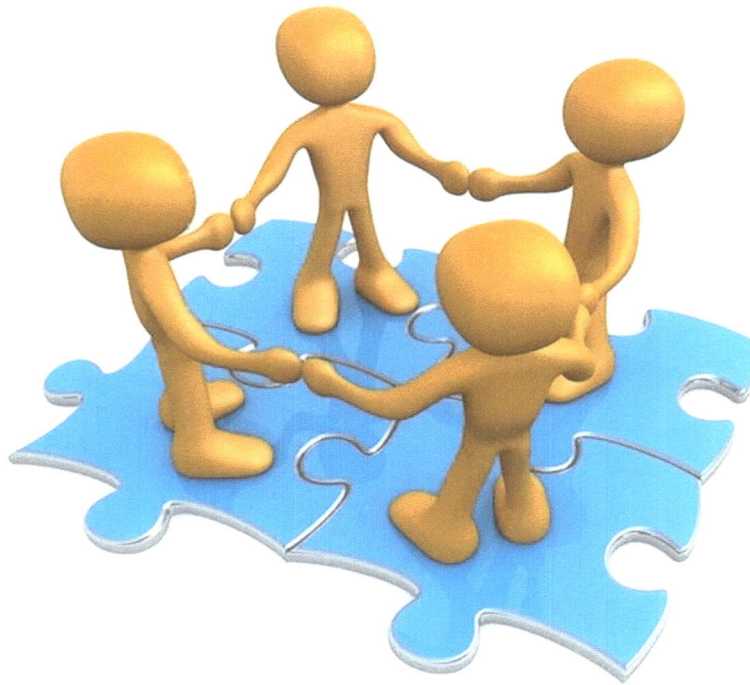

SESSION SEVEN

Connect Supporting the Primary Caregiver with the
Family Members "Roles and Responsibilities"

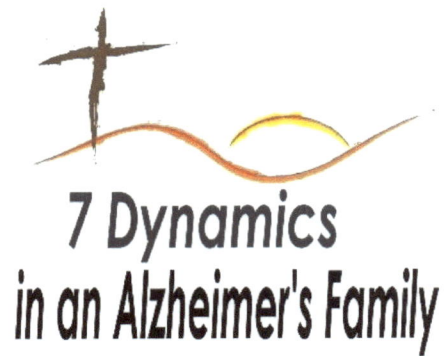

7 Dynamics
in an Alzheimer's Family

7th Dynamic

Assigning Family Members
Roles & Responsibilities

"My child, help your father in his old age, and don't give him grief during his life. 13 And if his understanding fails, be tolerant, and don't shame him, because you have all your faculties. 14 Taking care of one's father won't be forgotten. It will be credited to you against your sins." (Sirach 3:12–14).

God's plan has always been; that inside a family we are accountable to each other.

WHAT ARE ROLES AND RESPONSIBLITIES

Family Roles Matter:

An act of Love is when one picks up a Role and its Responsibilities. Given that over 60% of families fall apart during this journey, the odds for this happening when roles are clearly defined, communication and outlined, where everyone contributes, will reduce the percentage of failing for your family.

Assigning Roles

Think of a "Role" as being a category or character in a play. It is your part to be accountable for performing your assigned role each week. To do this a plan is needed.

It is for this reason that we will take the time to allocate the work load of primary caregiver to all those members of the family. Everyone has a role to play, in fact we have always had a role to play in our families, it was just rarely pointed out and written down on paper.

In this section, we will identify our roles and what area each of us will take responsibility for doing in the support of the family.

CREATING A "PLAN OF ACTION" Roles Assignments:

I. Who
II. Will Be Responsible to oversee What
III. How it will be done.
IV. Determine what resources are needed.
V. When it will be completed
VI. Report to family the progress.

The primary goal of the roles and responsibilities is to take these off the role of the Primary Caregiver, also to use the gifts and talents that are available from within the family. Our gifts have been given to us by God, and we are to use and share them with others.

By assigning "Other Chores" to the family member, a great burden will be lifted from the primary caregiver as they attend to the daily (hourly) needs of your loved one.

*DEESCRIPTION: The **Financial Role** is one of a company CFO, Accountant. The affairs of the estate would be included to this role and probate documents for timely court review processing. Include to this list month budgets and bills paying, managing financial investments and insurances.*

ROLES: _____

    A.   Tasks that involve all of the loved one's financial affairs.

    B.   Tasks that involve the loved one's real estate property.

    C.   Tasks that involve the loved one's possessions above a stated dollar amount.

    D.   Decision participation in affairs involving expenses, past and projected.

    E.   Monitoring and reporting the cost of living budget, medical bills follow up on payments.

    F.   Matters of Insurances.

    G. Matters of debt collection responses and planning.

    H. Matters of receivables in payments, interest, earning, promissory notes, etc.

    I.   Matters of personal property

    J.   OTHER: _____

*DESCRIPTION: The **Legal Secretary Role** is one of coordinating the legal aspect of the loved ones estate and personal care, completing, processing and filing of documents.*

ROLE: _____

A. Tasks that involve the loved one's legal affairs.

B. Tasks that involve the loved ones legal responsibly for real estate Property.

C. Tasks that involve the loved one's legal possessions above a state dollar amount.

D. Decision participation in affairs involving healthcare from a legal perspective,

E. Identifying all past and projected issues of the loved one and their legal accountabilities.

F. Monitoring and reporting the status of all legal affairs as it is related to their living budget, medical bills,

    monthly bills and financial interest.

G. Matters of Insurances and investments from a legal perspective.

H. Matters of debt collection responses and planning from a legal perspective.

I. Matters of receivables in payments, interest, earning, promissory notes, etc. from a legal perspective.

J. Matters of personal property from a legal perspective

K. OTHER: _____

*DESCRIPTION: The **Medical Records Organizer** Role is one of a organizer of records and health related documents for the loved one.*

ROLES: _____

    A.   Tasks that involve the loved one's medical affairs documents, appointments and communication with medical teams.

    B.   Tasks that involve the loved ones Medical Health Records.

    C.   Tasks that involve the loved one's appointment preparations.

    D.   Communicating the facts for decision making participation in affairs involving health and medical services. Knowing the labs, diagnosis test results, pharmacy drug interactions and side effects, allergies.

    E.   Monitoring and reporting the outcome of tests results and follow up plan of treatments. To do the research on these tests and communicate the facts.

    F.   Assist in getting to and from appointments.

    G.   Updating the Medical Records Binder.

    H.   OTHER: _____

let us remember that with God nothing is impossible; and as we read and hear his promises, let us turn them into prayers, Luke 1:38, *"I am the Lord's servant; let it be done unto me according to thy word"*.

In our roles and responsibilities as a family member, we are care-partners, we are here to be the servant of the Lord in the journey of our loved one and their primary caregiver, both physically and spiritually.

*DESCRIPTION: The **Support Network Coordination** Role is one of a company CFO, Accountant. The affairs of the estate would be included to this role and probate documents for time court review processing.,*

Roles: _____

A. Tasks that involve the loved one's support network from the community and family.

B. Tasks that involve the loved one's immediate family communication link, frequency and quality of check in and being compassionate.

C. Organizes family meetings or skype conference calls.

D. Tasks that involve the loved one's family and associations, parish volunteer positions.

E. Tasks that involve allowing the primary caregiver to participate in outside activities of their choosing.

F. Coordinating the friends and support groups for the primary caregiver.

G. Home Health Aid and Respite services for the primary caregivers support.

H. Mail Order Medical Supply's and mail order pharmacy coordination.

I. House Cleaning Service

J. Address all Yard and House Maintenance issues.

K. Issues of safety in the home and home security.

L. Getting to and from appointments for both the loved one and the primary caregiver.

M. Making sure the primary care giver has time and space for personal excerise, grooming needs, and time away from the house each week.

N. OTHER: _____

*DESCRIPTION: The **Spirituality Coordinator** Role is one ensuring the spirituality needs of the loved one and primary caregiver are available and being met with an adequate degree of support.*

Roles: _____

A. Tasks that involve ensuring the loved one and primary caregiver receive communion (the eucharist) on a regular bases.

B. Tasks that involve coordinating praying together, loved one, primary caregiver, family members. (out of state can be included by speaker phone, on a regular bases.

C. Tasks that involve the loved one and caregiver are given a break from each other, filled with spiritual exercise for each.

D. Matters of the sacraments response and planning.

E. OTHER: _____

Each Role has its own Responsibility. From the role assignment, the family member takes on that set of responsibilities, which each family member then creates their "Plan of Action" and this is how accountability is created.

The plan itself creates transparency that identifies where others can provide their assistance in helping to meet the family needs.

A "Plan of Action" is also a communication tool. This plan will identify your intentions for completing your responsibility.

CREATING A "PLAN OF ACTION":

1. WHO

2. Will DO WHAT

3. HOW IT WILL BE DONE

4. WHAT REASOURCES ARE NEEDED

5. WHEN IT WILL BE COMPLETED

The primary goal of the roles and responsibilities is to take these off the role of the Primary Caregiver, also to use the gifts and talents that are available from within the family.

By assigning "Other Chores" to the family member a great burden will be lifted from the primary caregiver as they attend to the daily (hourly) needs of your loved one.

 # 1 Financial Responsibilities: Assigned To: _____

Gather and organize financial documents in one place. Then, carefully review all documents, even if you're already familiar with them.

- Paying bills

- Arranging for benefit claims

- Making investment decisions

- Preparing tax returns

Financial documents include:

- Bank and brokerage account information

- Deeds, mortgage papers or ownership statements

- Insurance policies

- Monthly or outstanding bills

- Pension and other retirement benefit summaries (including VA benefits, if applicable)

- Rental income paperwork

- Social Security payment information

- Stock and bond certificates

Website for more details in managing someone else's money:
http://www.consumerfinance.gov/blog/managing-someone-elses-money/

Paying For Care: (managing bills)
A number of financial resources may be available to help cover the costs of care for the person Alzheimer's Disease or other dementia. Some may apply now and others in the future.

1st Assignment: Become familiar with this web page.
https://www.alz.org/care/alzheimers-dementia-costs-paying-for-care.asp

3rd **Assignment** https://www.alz.org/care/alzheimers-dementia-financial-legal-planning.asp

 # 2 Legal Responsibilities: Assigned To: _____

Gather and organize Legal documents in one place. Then, carefully review all documents, even if you're already familiar with them.

- Trust documents

- Power of Attorney, Healthcare Power of Attorney

- Will's

- End of life instructions

- Burial Plot Purchase

- Insurance Policies

- Do Not Resuscitate orders

Real Estate documents include:

- Property Deeds Transfer Up Death

- Mortgagees or Promissory Notes

- Joint Ownership in Land or Property

Personal Property

- Appraisals

- Bank Safety Deposit Boxes

- Memberships and Subscriptions

- Automatic Payment Bank Withdrawls

- Website for more details in managing some ones else's legal affairs:

https://www.alz.org/national/documents/brochure_legalplans.pdf

Legal Issues in Care: (managing legal affairs)
A number of legal resources may be available to help cover the legal aspects of care for the person Alzheimer's Disease or other dementia. Some may apply now and others in the future.

1st Assignment: Become familiar with this web page.
https://www.nia.nih.gov/health/legal-and-financial-planning-people-alzheimers
 # 3 Medical Profile and Records Responsibilities: Assigned To: _____

Gather and organize medical documents in one place. Then, carefully review all documents, even if you're already familiar with them.

- Vital Information

- Visits to the Doctor

- Medication Log

- Medical Consultation Log

- Doctor Visit

- Medical Contacts

- Blood Sugar Tracker

- Symptoms Tracker

- Blood Pressure Log

- Family History

- Medical Release

- Dental Log

- Transformation: Before

- Transformation: After

- Body Measurements Chart

- Personal Measurements Charts

- Vitamin Intake

- Sleeping Log Journal

- Lab Results

- Emergency Room Visits

- Prescriptions

- Known allergies

- Plan of Treatment

Other Services documents include:

- Home Healthcare Agency work, PT, OT, Respiratory, Nursing, Medical Supplies, Medical Equipment.

- Assisted Living, Rehabilitation Center, Memory Care Unit.

- Hospital Stay documents

- Home Heath Aid Services

Website for more details in managing some ones else's medical records:

http://betterhealthwhileaging.net/tools-for-caregivers-keeping-organizing-medical-information/

Paying For Care: (managing bills)
A number of financial resources may be available to help cover the costs of care for the person Alzheimer's Disease or other dementia. Some may apply now and others in the future.

1st Assignment: Become familiar with this web page.
https://www.sarahtitus.com/medical-binder/

 # 4 Support Network Coordinator Responsibilities Assigned To: _____

Coordinate and Support the Support Network. Then, carefully review preparation for up coming events, and follow up with past events.

- As a family set up a support network

- As a family set up a support network strategy to work each week

- Determine the resources required to ensure the support network works

- Handle each participant in the network separately, measure if they are the right entity.

Other Responsibilities include:

- Confirm that Banks, investments, insurance, physicians, home health services, attorneys are all working in the best interest of your loved one.

- Challenge your church to stop by

- Set up and schedule friends to stop by

- Create a newsletter for updating the network, just the facts.

- Schedule respite outings, overnight breaks

Website for more details in managing someone else's money:
http://www.aplaceformom.com/blog/7-19-16-ways-caregivers-can-build-a-support-system/

Paying For Care: (managing bills)
1st Assignment: Become familiar with this web page.

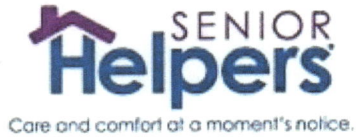

SENIOR
Helpers®
Care and comfort at a moment's notice.

STRONGSVILLE-PARMA
Call us today 234-542-2096
Click to see the surrounding area we serve

A list for a community support structure includes:

- Eldercare Attorney's
- Fiduciary Financial Advisors
- CPA Tax Accounts
- Insurance Brokers
- Realtor's (residential and commercial)
- Banker's
- Moving & Storage
- In Home Professional Organizer's
- Home Health Aid Companies
- Disposable Medical Supply and Medical Equipment Companies
- Medicare Advisor
- Veteran Service Officer
- Selecting a Memory Care Facility
- Physicians
- Nursing Homes
- Rehabilitation Centers
- Transportation Services
- Support Groups
- County, State and Federal aging services

 # 5 Spirituality Coordinator Responsibilities Assigned To: _____

Gather and organize financial documents in one place. Then, carefully review all documents, even if you're already familiar with them.

- Set up Homebound Eucharistic ministry

- Request prayer ministry to make home visit from parish

- Parish retreats for Caregiver and family members to attend together

- Driving to Mass, someone to watch loved one.

Other Responsibilities include:

- Once each month family gathers to pray rosary together

- Once a month Skype divine mercy chaplet, with family and invited support network

- First Saturday of the month morning Mass, blessed mother

- Monthly Adoration, 1 hour, someone to go, someone to stay and watch.

- Family Self-Directed Spiritual Development Program

- http://www.padrepiocleveland.org/   First Saturday each month communion with the Cleveland padre pio prayer group, starts with mass, the learning and prayer.

- Educate the family on how to use www.formed.org passcode 36TNDF.

- Educate the family on how to use http://www.usccb.org/bible/readings/Join a local "Legion of Mary" as an Auxiliary member. Look to a parish that has one.
- **Purchase from Amazon.com Dementia "Living in the memories of God" John Swinton. View video www.youtube: https://www.youtube.com/watch?v=AvVqhX7E0nU**

The _____ Role & Responsibility

CURRENT STATUS

What is the loved one's current stage?   _____

Recent Assessment Results? _____

Secondary Diagnosis?   _____

Required Action for Secondary Diagnosis to be addressed: (if any)

_____
_____
_____
_____
_____
_____
_____
_____

The Critical Issue to be addressed: (in this stage)

_____
_____
_____
_____
_____
_____
_____
_____

SECTION VI. CONCLUSION

By accepting the family structure as a channel of "Support" a wealth of resources have become available. When using the 7 Dynamics in an Alzheimer's Family to access this channel, more is gain out of what is done. In order to maximize the effectiveness of the Family Structure, accessing other support structures is needed. The 7 Dynamics in an Alzheimer's Family model is used with these support structure, too.

There are three other structures that a family needs to access in this journey:

1. Church Support Structure
2. Community Support Structure
3. Employer Support Structure

The three primary tasks of the Alzheimer's family:

1. Learn the 7 Dynamics in an Alzheimer's Family and how to use them.
2. Get the loved one's affairs in order, use The Alzheimer's Journey, It's Time to get Organized, written by Roy Poillon R~House Alzheimer's Family Learning Center.
3. Connecting the Puzzle Pieces is a five book series used to educate the Alzheimer's family from the vantage point of each separate stage of the disease progression. Connecting the Puzzle Pieces, written by Roy Poillon R~House Alzheimer's Family Learning Center.

R~ House
Alzheimer's Family Learning Center

7 Dynamics in an Alzheimer's Family

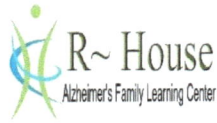

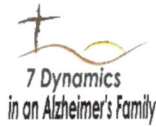

Educate and Train the Family

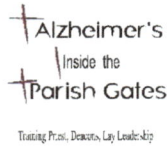

Alzheimer's Inside the Parish Gates

Training Priest, Deacons, Lay Leadership

Educate the Church Leaders and Staff

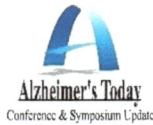

Alzheimer's Today

Conference & Symposium Update

Bring together the Community Support

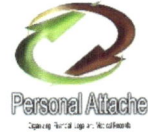

Personal Attache

Organize and Unite the Family

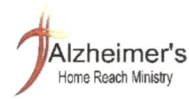

Alzheimer's Home Reach Ministry

Provide Church Ministry Outreach Model

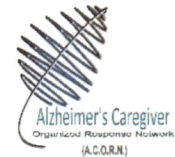

Alzheimer's Caregiver
Organized Response Network
(A.C.O.R.N.)

A "Wellness Health Plan Benefit" for Employer's

A Complete Response to Support the Alzheimer's Family

CONTACT US

R~HOUSE ALZHEIMER'S FAMILY LEARNING CENTERS OFFERS

1. On site learning center seminars (located in Cleveland, Ohio)

2. Parish or church seminars for organizations

3. Speaking engagement's

4. On-line seminars for families (using Go-To Meetings® web services) that are caring for a loved one with Alzheimer's disease.

TO SET UP A SEMINAR AT YOUR ORGANIZATION OR CHURCH

CONTACT US: (440) 385-7605

EMAIL: WITTSENDCONSULTING@GMAIL.COM

If you would like more information on starting an R~House Alzheimer's Family Learning Center in your area, contact us (440) 385-7605 email: wittsendconsulting@gmail.com

We also offer a turnkey model for an *"Alzheimer's Home Reach Ministry"*, to start from a parish or church Provide ministry to the Alzheimer's family at their home of nursing facility. Meet them where they are, as they are.

R~ House

Alzheimer's Family Learning Center

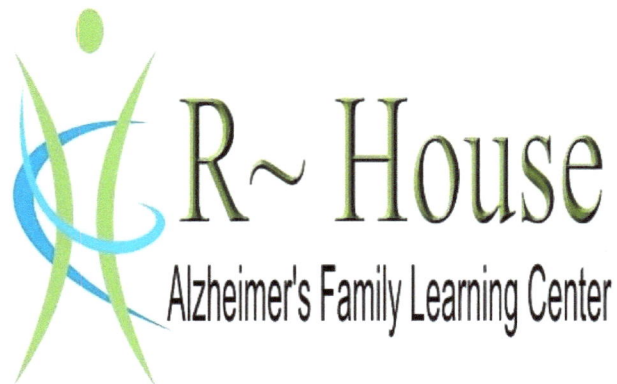

Contact us to lead your own "R~House Alzheimer's Family Learning Center" in your local community. We have all the materials needed to get you started.

440.385.7605